Copyright ©2015 Ferdinand H. Quinco

All rights reserved. No part of this publication may be reproduced, distributed, or transmitted in any form or by any means, including photocopying, recording, or other electronic or mechanical methods, without the prior written permission of the publisher, except in the case of brief quotations embodied in critical reviews and certain other noncommercial uses permitted by copyright law.

Contents

INTRODUCTION 4
CBD: THE MULTIPURPOSE MOLECULE 8
   HOW DOES CBD WORK 9
   THE ENDOCANNABINOID SYSTEM 10
   PHARMACEUTICAL CBD 11
CBD OIL 13
   Is CBD marijuana 14
   Where does CBD come from 14
   How CBD works 15
   Benefits and Uses of CBD Oil 15
   Are There Any Side Effects 24
   The Bottom Line 25
   THE CBD CHALLENGE 26
   WHAT ABOUT CBD FROM HEMP 27
Making Cannabis Oil 29
   All You Need To Know About Cannabis Oil 30
   Rick Simpson's Cannaoil Odyssey 31
   Rick simpsons cannabis oil 31
   How to Make CBD Oil At Home 35
   At Home CBD: You Get Back What You Put In 35
   The Simplest CBD Extraction Method: Using a Carrier Oil Solvent 37

The Science of At-Home CBD Extraction 38
Choosing Your Ingredients for At-Home CBD 38
Homemade CBD Oil 41
Conclusion 42
Different Ways on How to Make CBD Oil 42
Oil Method 42
Alcohol Method 44
The Different Ways to Use CBD Oil 45
Easy Steps 46
Making cannabis oil 2 49
How To Make Cannabis Oil At Home: Rick Simpson's Way .. 50
Cannabis Oil Applications 62
Topical Uses 62
Edible Uses 62
Summary 67
How to make cannabis oil for medical purposes 69
Tools and ingredients needed 70
Make the oil 70
Why make your own cannabis oil for medical purposes 71

INTRODUCTION

If you've been part of the cannabis community for any length of time, especially for medical purposes, you've likely heard a good deal about the therapeutic effects of CBD. Also known as cannabidiol, CBD is a cannabinoid with anti-inflammatory, analgesic, and anxiolytic effects. It can treat chronic pain and inflammation, regulate mood and sleep, ease nausea, and treat seizures and muscle spasms, just to name a few applications.

There is an overwhelming abundance of retailers selling CBD oil on the open market, but it can be hard to determine the quality and purity of the product you're buying. Unless you're buying from a trusted retailer (see our CBD Buyer's Guide to learn what to look for when buying CBD), sorting out the good products from the junk can be difficult.

You can skip the guesswork by making CBD yourself, in the comfort and privacy of your own home, with no special equipment or toxic chemicals. This way, you control every step of the process, from selecting the strain to choosing the dosage concentration, to the actual extraction itself; you know exactly what you're getting in the finished product and can modify your materials or methods according to your specific needs. It might seem complicated, but we promise you, you can do this! Here, we'll discuss the science of cannabinoid extraction and tell you how to make CBD oil at home for yourself.

Cannabis oil is a potent substance that can be eaten, inhaled, or rubbed on topically. It is the foundation to many tasty edible marijuana recipes. The THC content in the oil brings on an enjoyable psychoactive effect when ingested, so it's a great base for chocolate brownies!

Cannabis oil is also a potent medicine containing large amounts of healthy cannabinoids. The two cannabinoids with the strongest medicinal value are THC and CBD. Both are present in a well made cannabis oil. The oil can be used to treat a whole host of physiological and psychological conditions, including headache, insomnia, muscle pain, inflammation, arthritis, glaucoma, anxiety and depression. Cannabis oil can even have anti-cancer effects. Studies are suggesting that cannabinoids can inhibit tumor growth by disrupting the formation of new blood vessels that the tumors need to grow. Cannabinoids even seem to attack cancerous cells while leaving healthy cells intact. Go cannabinoids!

Using cannabis oil is a very effective way to get a high dose of health-promoting cannabinoids, because the refining process removes all of the plant material and leaves only pure oil behind. This oil contains high levels of THC and CBD, so it's possible to consume higher doses of the healthy cannabinoids than if you smoke your medical cannabis.

It is definitely advisable to choose a high-quality strain of medical marijuana to make your cannabis oil with. If you have a cannabis card you can ask at your local dispensary which strain they recommend for making a nice and pure oil, or you can grow your own weed at home and use that. It is good to use an organic strain because otherwise the unpleasant chemical fertilizers and pesticides that are used in the growing process in some 420 card states will end up in your oil in concentrated levels. The purer the strain, the better.

It is important that you choose the right location to make your oil. You will need to find a well-ventilated and open space with windows and a gas or electric stove.

Cannabidiol (CBD) is a naturally occurring compound found in the resinous flower of cannabis, a plant with a rich history as a medicine going back thousands of years. Today the therapeutic properties of CBD are being tested and confirmed by scientists and doctors around the world. A safe, non-addictive substance, CBD is one of more than a hundred "phytocannabinoids," which are unique to cannabis and endow the plant with its robust therapeutic profile.

CBD is closely related to another important medicinally active phytocannabinoid: tetrahydrocannabinol (THC), the compound that causes the high that cannabis is famous for. These are the two components of cannabis that have been most studied by scientists.

Both CBD and THC have significant therapeutic attributes. But unlike THC, CBD does not make a person feel "stoned" or intoxicated. That's because CBD and THC act in different ways on different receptors in the brain and body.

CBD can actually lessen or neutralize the psychoactive effects of THC, depending on how much of each compound is consumed. Many people want the health benefits of cannabis without the high - or with less of a high.

The fact that CBD is therapeutically potent as well as non-intoxicating, and easy to take as a CBD oil, makes it an appealing treatment option for those who are cautious about trying cannabis for the first time.

CBD: THE MULTIPURPOSE MOLECULE

Many people are seeking alternatives to pharmaceuticals with harsh side effects – medicine more in synch with natural processes. By tapping into how we function biologically on a deep level, CBD can provide relief for chronic pain, anxiety, inflammation, depression and many other conditions.

Extensive scientific research - much of it sponsored by the U.S. government - and mounting anecdotal accounts from patients and physicians highlight CBD's potential as a treatment for a wide range of maladies, including (but not limited to):

- Autoimmune diseases (inflammation, rheumatoid arthritis)
- Neurological conditions (Alzheimer's, dementia, Parkinson's, multiple sclerosis, epilepsy, Huntington's chorea, stroke, traumatic brain injury)
- Metabolic syndrome (diabetes, obesity)
- Neuropsychiatric illness (autism, ADHD, PTSD, alcoholism)
- Gut disorders (colitis, Crohn's)
- Cardiovascular dysfunction (atherosclerosis, arrhythmia)
- Skin disease (acne, dermatitis, psoriasis)

CBD has proven neuroprotective effects and its anti-cancer properties are being investigated at several academic research centers in the United States and elsewhere. A 2010 brain cancer study by California scientists found that CBD "enhances the inhibitory effects of THC on human glioblastoma cell proliferation and survival." This means that CBD makes THC even more potent as an anticancer substance. Also in 2010, German researchers reported that CBD stimulates neurogenesis, the growth of new brain cells, in adult mammals.

HOW DOES CBD WORK

CBD and THC interact with our bodies in a variety of ways. One of the main ways they impact us is by mimicking and augmenting the effects of the compounds in our bodies called "endogenous cannabinoids" - so named because of their similarity to the compounds found in the cannabis plant. These "endocannabinoids" are part of a regulatory system called the "endocannabinoid system".

The discovery of the endocannabinoid system has significantly advanced our understanding of health and disease. It has major implications for nearly every area of medical science and helps to explain how and why CBD and THC are such versatile compounds - and why cannabis is such a widely consumed mood-altering plant, despite its illegal status.

THE ENDOCANNABINOID SYSTEM

The endocannabinoid system plays a crucial role in regulating a broad range of physiological processes that affect our everyday experience - our mood, our energy level, our intestinal fortitude, immune activity, blood pressure, bone density, glucose metabolism, how we experience pain, stress, hunger, and more.

What happens if the endocannabinoid system doesn't function properly? What are the consequences of a chronically deficient or overactive endocannabinoid system?

In a word, disease.

Cutting-edge science has shown that the endocannabinoid system is dysregulated in nearly all pathological conditions. Thus, it stands to reason that "modulating endocannabinoid system activity may have therapeutic potential in almost all diseases affecting humans," as Pal Pacher and George Kunos, scientists with the U.S. National Institutes of Health (NIH), suggested in a 2014 publication. By modulating the endocannabinoid system and enhancing endocannabinoid tone, CBD and THC can slow or in some cases stop disease progression.

PHARMACEUTICAL CBD

There's a lot of excitement about the healing potential of CBD - with good reason.

But it wasn't until June 25, 2018, that the U.S. Food and Drug Administration (FDA) recognized cannabidiol as a real medicine by approving Epidiolex, an almost pure pharmaceutical CBD formulation, as a treatment for two severe pediatric seizure disorders, Lennox-Gastaut syndrome and Dravet syndrome.

This was the first time since the peak of the reefer madness era 80 years ago - when "marihuana" became a crime instead of a cure that the federal government had given an official thumbs-up for a cannabis-derived product.

In response to the FDA's historic decision, the Drug Enforcement Administration (DEA) announced in September 2018 that it had removed Epidiolex from Schedule I classification, a category reserved for dangerous drugs with no medical value. Henceforth, Epidiolex would be considered a Schedule V drug, the least dangerous designation under the Controlled Substances Act.

But the DEA kept cannabis and CBD itself on Schedule I as an illegal narcotic. In the world according to Uncle Sam, pharmaceutical CBD is officially the only good cannabinoid while the rest of the plant remains an 'evil' weed.

Given CBD's reputation as a popular, artisanal remedy, one would think that Epidiolex would command a lot of "off label" attention. After all, physicians often prescribe pharmaceuticals off label to treat conditions that were not the actual focus of clinical trials. But the costly price tag for Epidiolex (more than $30,000 annually) precludes off label prescribing as well as affordable access for tens of millions of Americans without health insurance.

CBD OIL

For those who can't obtain pharmaceutical CBD, there are numerous internet storefronts, community markets, coffee shops, health clubs, chiropractic offices, upscale boutiques and gas stations that retail various hemp-derived CBD oil products, including pure CBD isolates comparable in chemical make-up to Epidiolex.

CBD oil products and flower with varying levels of THC and CBD are also available for smoking or vaping at cannabis dispensaries in states that have legalized the herb for therapeutic use.

In response to massive consumer demand, a huge, unregulated market in CBD oil products reached a critical mass in 2018. A surge of consumer interest in all things CBD was suddenly newsworthy with hosanas of praise coming from athletes, film stars, soccer moms, and parents of desperately ill children.

CBD oil has been touted as a curative for the sick and a preventive for the healthy, an all-purpose palliative for pets as well as people of all ages.

But along with a growing awareness of cannabidiol as a potential health aide, there has also been a proliferation of misconceptions about CBD and cannabis therapeutics.

Is CBD marijuana

CBD oil may have a number of health benefits. Until recently, the best-known compound in cannabis was delta-9 tetrahydrocannabinol (THC). This is the most active ingredient in marijuana. Marijuana contains both THC and CBD, and these compounds have different effects. THC creates a mind-altering "high" when a person smokes it or uses it in cooking. This is because THC breaks down when we apply heat and introduce it into the body.

CBD is different. Unlike THC, it is not psychoactive. This means that CBD does not change a person's state of mind when they use it. However, CBD does appear to produce significant changes in the body, and some research suggests that it has medical benefits.

Where does CBD come from

The least processed form of the cannabis plant is hemp. Hemp contains most of the CBD that people use medicinally. Hemp and marijuana come from the same plant, Cannabis sativa, but the two are very different.

Over the years, marijuana farmers have selectively bred their plants to contain high levels of THC and other compounds that interested them, often because the compounds produced a smell or had another effect on the plant's flowers.

However, hemp farmers have rarely modified the plant. These hemp plants are used to create CBD oil.

How CBD works

All cannabinoids, including CBD, produce effects in the body by attaching to certain receptors. The human body produces certain cannabinoids on its own. It also has two receptors for cannabinoids, called the CB1 receptors and CB2 receptors. CB1 receptors are present throughout the body, but many are in the brain.

The CB1 receptors in the brain deal with coordination and movement, pain, emotions, and mood, thinking, appetite, and memories, and other functions. THC attaches to these receptors. CB2 receptors are more common in the immune system. They affect inflammation and pain.

Researchers once believed that CBD attached to these CB2 receptors, but it now appears that CBD does not attach directly to either receptor. Instead, it seems to direct the body to use more of its own cannabinoids.

Benefits and Uses of CBD Oil

Cannabidiol is a popular natural remedy used for many common ailments.

Better known as CBD, it is one of the 104 chemical compounds known as cannabinoids found in the cannabis or marijuana plant, Cannabis sativa.

Tetrahydrocannabinol (THC) is the main psychoactive cannabinoid found in cannabis, and causes the sensation of getting "high" that's often associated with marijuana. However, unlike THC, CBD is not psychoactive. This quality makes CBD an appealing option for those who are looking for relief from pain and other symptoms without the mind-altering effects of marijuana or certain pharmaceutical drugs.

CBD oil is made by extracting CBD from the cannabis plant, then diluting it with a carrier oil like coconut or hemp seed oil. It's gaining momentum in the health and wellness world, with some scientific studies confirming it may help treat a variety of ailments like chronic pain and anxiety.

Here are seven health benefits of CBD oil that are backed by scientific evidence.

1. Can Relieve Pain

Marijuana has been used to treat pain as far back as 2900 B.C. More recently, scientists have discovered that certain components of marijuana, including CBD, are responsible for its pain-relieving effects.

The human body contains a specialized system called the endocannabinoid system (ECS), which is involved in regulating a variety of functions including sleep, appetite, pain and immune system response.

The body produces endocannabinoids, which are neurotransmitters that bind to cannabinoid receptors in your nervous system.

Studies have shown that CBD may help reduce chronic pain by impacting endocannabinoid receptor activity, reducing inflammation and interacting with neurotransmitters. For example, one study in rats found that CBD injections reduced pain response to surgical incision, while another rat study found that oral CBD treatment significantly reduced sciatic nerve pain and inflammation. Several human studies have found that a combination of CBD and THC is effective in treating pain related to multiple sclerosis and arthritis.

An oral spray called Sativex, which is a combination of THC and CBD, is approved in several countries to treat pain related to multiple sclerosis. In a study of 47 people with multiple sclerosis, those treated with Sativex for one month experienced a significant improvement in pain, walking and muscle spasms, compared to the placebo group.

Another study found that Sativex significantly improved pain during movement, pain at rest and sleep quality in 58 people with rheumatoid arthritis.

2. Could Reduce Anxiety and Depression

Anxiety and depression are common mental health disorders that can have devastating impacts on health and well-being. According to the World Health Organization, depression is the single largest contributor to disability worldwide, while anxiety disorders are ranked sixth.

Anxiety and depression are usually treated with pharmaceutical drugs, which can cause a number of side effects including drowsiness, agitation, insomnia, sexual dysfunction and headache.

What's more, medications like benzodiazepines can be addictive and may lead to substance abuse. CBD oil has shown promise as a treatment for both depression and anxiety, leading many who live with these disorders to become interested in this natural approach. In one study, 24 people with social anxiety disorder received either 600 mg of CBD or a placebo before a public speaking test. The group that received the CBD had significantly less anxiety, cognitive impairment and discomfort in their speech performance, compared to the placebo group.

CBD oil has even been used to safely treat insomnia and anxiety in children with post-traumatic stress disorder. CBD has also shown antidepressant-like effects in several animal studies. These qualities are linked to CBD's ability to act on the brain's receptors for serotonin, a neurotransmitter that regulates mood and social behavior.

3. Can Alleviate Cancer-Related Symptoms

CBD may help reduce symptoms related to cancer and side effects related to cancer treatment, like nausea, vomiting and pain.

One study looked at the effects of CBD and THC in 177 people with cancer-related pain who did not experience relief from pain medication.

Those treated with an extract containing both compounds experienced a significant reduction in pain compared to those who received only THC extract.

CBD may also help reduce chemotherapy-induced nausea and vomiting, which are among the most common chemotherapy-related side effects for those with cancer. Though there are drugs that help with these distressing symptoms, they are sometimes ineffective, leading some people to seek alternatives.

A study of 16 people undergoing chemotherapy found that a one-to-one combination of CBD and THC administered via mouth spray reduced chemotherapy-related nausea and vomiting better than standard treatment alone.Some test-tube and animal studies have even shown that CBD may have anticancer properties. For example, one test-tube study found that concentrated CBD induced cell death in human breast cancer cells. Another study showed that CBD inhibited the spread of aggressive breast cancer cells in mice.

However, these are test-tube and animal studies, so they can only suggest what might work in people. More studies in humans are needed before conclusions can be made.

4. May Reduce Acne

Acne is a common skin condition that affects more than 9% of the population.It is thought to be caused by a number of factors, including genetics, bacteria, underlying inflammation and the overproduction of sebum, an oily secretion made by sebaceous glands in the skin.

Based on recent scientific studies, CBD oil may help treat acne due to its anti-inflammatory properties and ability to reduce sebum production. One test-tube study found that CBD oil prevented sebaceous gland cells from secreting excessive sebum, exerted anti-inflammatory actions and prevented the activation of "pro-acne" agents like inflammatory cytokines.

Another study had similar findings, concluding that CBD may be an efficient and safe way to treat acne, thanks in part to its remarkable anti-inflammatory qualities. Though these results are promising, human studies exploring the effects of CBD on acne are needed.

5. Might Have Neuroprotective Properties

Researchers believe that CBD's ability to act on the endocannabinoid system and other brain signaling systems may provide benefits for those with neurological disorders. In fact, one of the most studied uses for CBD is in treating neurological disorders like epilepsy and multiple sclerosis. Though research in this area is still relatively new, several studies have shown promising results.

Sativex, an oral spray consisting of CBD and THC, has been proven to be a safe and effective way to reduce muscle spasticity in people with multiple sclerosis.

One study found that Sativex reduced spasms in 75% of 276 people with multiple sclerosis who were experiencing muscle spasticity that was resistant to medications.

Another study gave 214 people with severe epilepsy 0.9–2.3 grams of CBD oil per pound (2–5 g/kg) of body weight. Their seizures reduced by a median of 36.5%.

One more study found that CBD oil significantly reduced seizure activity in children with Dravet syndrome, a complex childhood epilepsy disorder, compared to a placebo. However, it's important to note that some people in both these studies experienced adverse reactions associated with CBD treatment, such as convulsions, fever and diarrhea.

CBD has also been researched for its potential effectiveness in treating several other neurological diseases. For example, several studies have shown that treatment with CBD improved quality of life and sleep quality for people with Parkinson's disease.

Additionally, animal and test-tube studies have shown that CBD may decrease inflammation and help prevent the neurodegeneration associated with Alzheimer's disease.

In one long-term study, researchers gave CBD to mice genetically predisposed to Alzheimer's disease, finding that it helped prevent cognitive decline.

6. Could Benefit Heart Health

Recent research has linked CBD with several benefits for the heart and circulatory system, including the ability to lower high blood pressure. High blood pressure is linked to higher risks of a number of health conditions, including stroke, heart attack and metabolic syndrome.

Studies indicate that CBD may be a natural and effective treatment for high blood pressure. One recent study treated 10 healthy men with one dose of 600 mg of CBD oil and found it reduced resting blood pressure, compared to a placebo. The same study also gave the men stress tests that normally increase blood pressure. Interestingly, the single dose of CBD led the men to experience a smaller blood pressure increase than normal in response to these tests.

Researchers have suggested that the stress- and anxiety-reducing properties of CBD are responsible for its ability to help lower blood pressure. Additionally, several animal studies have demonstrated that CBD may help reduce the inflammation and cell death associated with heart disease due to its powerful antioxidant and stress-reducing properties. For example, one study found that treatment with CBD reduced oxidative stress and prevented heart damage in diabetic mice with heart disease.

7. Several Other Potential Benefits

CBD has been studied for its role in treating a number of health issues other than those outlined above. Though more studies are needed, CBD is thought to provide the following health benefits:

- Antipsychotic effects: Studies suggest that CBD may help people with schizophrenia and other mental disorders by reducing psychotic symptoms.
- Substance abuse treatment: CBD has been shown to modify circuits in the brain related to drug addiction. In rats, CBD has been shown to reduce morphine dependence and heroin-seeking behavior.
- Anti-tumor effects: In test-tube and animal studies, CBD has demonstrated anti-tumor effects. In animals, it has been shown to prevent the spread of breast, prostate, brain, colon and lung cancer.
- Diabetes prevention: In diabetic mice, treatment with CBD reduced the incidence of diabetes by 56% and significantly reduced inflammation.

Are There Any Side Effects

Though CBD is generally well tolerated and considered safe, it may cause adverse reactions in some people. Side effects noted in studies include:

- Diarrhea
- Changes in appetite
- Fatigue

CBD is also known to interact with several medications. Before you start using CBD oil, discuss it with your doctor to ensure your safety and avoid potentially harmful interactions.

The Bottom Line

CBD oil has been studied for its potential role in treating many common health issues, including anxiety, depression, acne and heart disease. For those with cancer, it may even provide a natural alternative for pain and symptom relief.

Research on the potential health benefits of CBD oil is ongoing, so new therapeutic uses for this natural remedy are sure to be discovered. Though there is much to be learned about the efficacy and safety of CBD, results from recent studies suggest that CBD may provide a safe, powerful natural treatment for many health issues.

THE CBD CHALLENGE

CBD is a molecule, not a miracle. Many people could benefit significantly from legal access to a wide range of cannabis remedies, not just low-THC or no-THC products. CBD alone may not always do the trick. There is compelling evidence that CBD works best in combination with THC and the full spectrum of other cannabis components.

Figuring out how to optimize one's therapeutic use of cannabis is the driving force behind the great laboratory experiment in democracy known as medical marijuana that's been unfolding state-by-state and country-by-country in recent years.

The advent of potent cannabis oil concentrates, non-intoxicating CBD-rich products, and innovative, smokeless delivery systems has transformed the therapeutic landscape and changed the public conversation about cannabis.

It's no longer a matter of debating whether cannabis has merit as an herbal medication - today the key challenge is discerning how to utilize cannabis for maximum therapeutic benefit. Given its low-risk profile, many people are using CBD as an add-on therapy to their existing treatment plans.

But most health professionals know little about CBD or cannabis therapeutics and they lack sufficient expertise to adequately counsel patients regarding dosage, modes of administration, CBD/THC synergies, and any risk factors, including interactions with other drugs.

Instead, the onus has been on a loose-knit community of self-reliant patients, supportive families and a few pioneer physicians who've learned a lot through trial and error and shared information about how to navigate promising avenues of cannabis therapy.

WHAT ABOUT CBD FROM HEMP

What began as a grassroots populist rebellion against cannabis prohibition would morph into a multibillion-dollar market catalyzed by the rediscovery of CBD as a wellness option. CBD oil is red hot and it seems that everyone - do-gooders as well as profiteers – wants a piece of the action.

CBD has also catalyzed the rebirth of the U.S. hemp industry, which lay dormant for decades because of drug war politics. The 2018 Farm Bill includes a provision that legalizes the cultivation of hemp (cannabis with less than 0.3 percent THC) in large part because of the popularity and driving economic force of CBD.

Growing hemp is now a legitimate agricultural enterprise in the United States. But extracting CBD-rich oil from hemp biomass and marketing CBD oil concentrates and isolates for ingestion and inhalation steps on Big Pharma's toes and is frowned upon by the DEA and the FDA.

Legalities aside, hemp-derived cannabidiol is just a mouse click or a phone tap away for anyone willing to roll the dice and purchase CBD oil products that are manufactured with little regulatory oversight.

The upside of all this is easy access to CBD oil; the downside is inconsistent quality.

Many hemp-derived CBD oil products are mislabeled as to cannabidiol and THC content. And poorly processed CBD oil may be tainted with toxic solvent residues, pesticides, corn syrup, artificial flavors and colors, and other contaminants.

Fortunately, good quality CBD oil products are also available for the conscientious consumer - the label reader, the brand researcher - who understands that cannabis and CBD are best used as part of a healthy lifestyle.

Making Cannabis Oil

We are literally living in the Golden Age of cannabis. There are so many different products it can be difficult to choose which to use...or even which to try first. From gummies to blunts to tinctures to creams, you can get your marijuana in any and every shape and form.

On one end, you've got your well-known methods of consumption, like joints and bongs. On the other end, you've got your lesser-known forms of cannabis, like live resin and cannabis oil. It's this latter form of cannabis — cannabis oil to which we'll devote our attention today.

Cannabis oil has been growing in popularity recently thanks to its ability to stop the growth of, and even destroy, cancer cells. It has other powerful medicinal effects (as you'll see below), but its anti-tumoral properties are the thing that gets most people excited.

In this book, we'll teach you how to make cannabis oil for yourself. That way, you can take advantage of all the healing without spending an arm and a leg. But before we get to the how-to, let's take a moment and learn what cannabis oil is and what it isn't.

All You Need To Know About Cannabis Oil

Cannabis oil is a special type of marijuana concentrate that has saved and improved countless lives. Cannabis oil is essentially pure THC or CBD which can be consumed in much larger doses than is possible by smoking, vaporizing, or ingesting raw cannabis flower.

Cannabis oil, to be clear, is not the same thing as CBD oil. Do not buy CBD or hemp oils online. Such products are often produced from industrial grade hemp which lacks the critical anticancer THC cannabinoid. The industrial hemp used in these bogus medications is also often grown with harsh, inorganic chemical fertilizers as opposed to organic marijuana.

"The only way to know that you have the real thing is to produce the proper oil yourself" according to none other than the Obi Wan Kenobi of Cannabis Oil, Rick Simpson himself.

We'll summarize Simpson's cannabis-oil-making process into simple steps that any stoner will be able to follow. We'll also share some of his sage advice for treating skin diseases, proper dosing, and his tips for ingesting the oil.

Rick Simpson's Cannaoil Odyssey

Rick Simpson's story is one of those modern-day miracles that we've all heard, but don't know whether to believe or not. We're here to tell you that this one is true. Mr. Simpson survived a severe head injury as well as skin cancer using only cannabis oil that he made himself at home.

His story has created so much public interest in the reefer oil remedy that the term "Rick Simpson Oil" is now synonymous with cannabis oil itself. Simpson first learned how THC reduced brain tumors in mice from a radio show that was discussing the results of a study from the University of Virginia two years after he witnessed his cousin die from cancer.

Rick simpsons cannabis oil

Rick Simpson's own difficulties started when he was using a highly-toxic aerosol spray to cover asbestos in a boiler room. The chemical was so powerful it caused his nervous system to shut down temporarily. He fell backward off his ladder and smashed his head on a protruding steel ring from a pipe.

Fortunately, Simpson doesn't recall any of this. But when he came to, "[He] was hung up in the pipes by the side of the boiler." He managed to make it down from the pipes to his office but was too disoriented to use the phone to call for help. A coworker took him to the hospital when he came in to start his shift.

Simpson suffered from crippling head pain and a constant ringing in his ears for an entire year when he learned more about medicinal marijuana from an episode of Dr. David Suzuki's The Nature of Things. Simpson tried pot even though his doctor wouldn't prescribe it to him and it helped.

Simpson wasn't fully recovered from his head trauma though. He was still a "chemical zombie." He wanted legal access to medical marijuana as well, so Simpson asked his doctor if he would prescribe it to him as an essential oil. His doctor still refused to prescribe him cannabis.

Simpson's doctor did agree, however, that taking a marijuana oil extraction seemed like a better medicinal way of using cannabis compared to smoking it. Simpson's doctor also told him that they had exhausted every possible treatment for his head trauma.

That's when Mr. Simpson started making his own cannabis oil. "Once the system gave up on me, I just continued making oil and taking it on a regular basis. The ringing was still there, but now I could live with it. Within a few months, people saw the difference. The oil controlled the pain, my blood pressure, and it allowed me to sleep. I lost weight and looked 20 years younger."

Simpson began crossing swords with the medical establishment again in 2003 after his doctor surgically removed what turned out to be a patch of cancerous skin that was growing near Simpson's eye.

Simpson recalled the radio report he listened to about cannabis killing cancer tumors in mice after he took the bandage off the red, infected, pussing patch of skin the doctor had removed. Simpson felt compelled to dab some of his oil on the cancerous spot. He also put some of his oil on band-aids and covered the two other cancerous skin growths on his face and chest.

"Four days later, I took the band-aids off and both bumps had disappeared," Simpson says. The growth near his eye returned a few weeks later, but Simpson simply reapplied more of his oil and his skin completely healed after another four days.

Simpson could hardly wait to share the discovery with his doctor who had been completely reluctant to prescribe pot for Simpson's head trauma. Simpson told his doctor's wife and receptionist. "I treated my skin cancers with hemp oil" he began.

But he'd barely gotten the words "hemp oil" out, he recalls, before the receptionist went ballistic: "The doctor will not go there!" she yelled. "The doctor will not prescribe this!"

Simpson, undaunted, applied his homemade "hemp oil" to his mother's weeping psoriasis and the sores and scales on her skin both cleared up and completely disappeared within a few weeks. "In the first year, I treated 50 to 60 people for various skin conditions," Simpson says.

In fact, he was able to help terminally-ill patients given only weeks to live, to survive and recover from stage four terminal cancer by ingesting the cannabis oil. Simpson estimates that about 70% of terminal cancer patients, the ones with the least amount of chemotherapy, are most likely to survive and recover from cancer using cannabis oil.

Rick Simpson has since treated thousands of patients in Canada. He cannot visit the United States since he was convicted of marijuana possession, cultivation, and trafficking in Canada in 2007. Rick Simpson still freely shares his secrets for making homemade cannabis oil online, however.

Simpson himself was thankfully only fined $2,000. He also didn't have to serve the twelve years of jail time he was facing since the judge determined that there was no criminal intent in the case and since the scientific evidence supported his claims.

How to Make CBD Oil At Home

You can skip the guesswork by making CBD yourself, in the comfort and privacy of your own home, with no special equipment or toxic chemicals. This way, you control every step of the process, from selecting the strain to choosing the dosage concentration, to the actual extraction itself; you know exactly what you're getting in the finished product and can modify your materials or methods according to your specific needs. It might seem complicated, but we promise you, you can do this! Here, we'll discuss the science of cannabinoid extraction and tell you how to make CBD oil at home for yourself.

At Home CBD: You Get Back What You Put In

First, we need to talk about choosing your starting material (aka the flower or extract you'll be infusing into the oil). This is what determines the cannabinoid content of your finished CBD oil (and therefore its effects on you). This is especially important when using the method we'll outline below, because it's not possible to extract only CBD without taking other cannabinoids, like THC, along for the ride. This means that if you start with a high-THC flower, you'll end up with a high-THC oil. There is no way to separate the THC from the CBD without specialized laboratory equipment. Therefore, depending on your starting material, your finished CBD oil may or may not also contain THC; it all depends on the cannabinoid content of your starting material.

You can absolutely use THC-rich strains of cannabis for your CBD oil if you choose. THC has a number of therapeutic benefits that may work in concert with those of CBD, producing synergistic effects. If you're going this route, we recommend an indica strain, as you'll get the benefits of high CBD and other beneficial cannabinoid content without the "head high" associated with sativas, which can make it hard to function for some consumers. This type of CBD oil (sometimes called Rick Simpson Oil, or RSO, in this high-THC incarnation) is especially good for patients suffering from severe chronic pain and various cancers. However, it can cause drowsiness and impairment at high doses so it may not be right for everyone.

So, what do you do if you want to make CBD oil with little-to-no THC? If you're fortunate enough to live in a state where cannabis is legal for you, you can request a high-CBD strain from your budtender at the dispensary; they'll gladly point you in the right direction. However, if you don't reside in a state where you can buy your flower from a trusted, licensed professional, Farm Bill-compliant hemp flower is legal for purchase, though it's not available over the counter in most places.

This means that it is legal to order organically-grown hemp flower in all fifty states, and you can then use this hemp flower to make your CBD oil. Since hemp contains 0.3% or less THC, you won't feel its effects, but you'll get all the benefits from the high CBD, CBN, CBG, and other non-psychoactive cannabinoids contained in the hemp flower. You could also use raw CBD oil (meaning it has not yet been infused into a carrier oil), like uncut CO2 oil, instead of the flowers or buds as the starting material.

If you're able, try smoking or vaping a little beforehand to get an idea of what its effects will be like before committing. Any adverse or undesirable effects will wear off within an hour or two this way, as opposed to up to eight hours for cannabinoids ingested orally.

The Simplest CBD Extraction Method: Using a Carrier Oil Solvent

The method we'll discuss here extracts cannabinoids (referred to as CBD from here on out for simplicity's sake) through an easy process that requires little skill and relatively little time spent standing over a pot. There is another, more complicated (and potentially dangerous) method using alcohol as a solvent, but we feel like that deserves its own article (it isn't for everyone), so we'll save it for another time. Here, we'll focus on a much more accessible method with fewer safety requirements: infusing CBD into a carrier oil.

The Science of At-Home CBD Extraction

This method works because CBD is soluble with nonpolar molecules, meaning it can't dissolve in water (a polar molecule), but can dissolve in fats (nonpolar) and alcohols (technically a polar molecule overall, but alcohol has a special ability to bond with nonpolar molecules in ways that water cannot—polarity is a spectrum, and while water is far off to one end, alcohol is close enough to the middle to, well, go both ways). This extraction method takes advantage of the lipid-solubility, or dissolvability in fats, of cannabinoids.

Choosing Your Ingredients for At-Home CBD

Using a carrier oil as your solvent we recommend MCT or coconut oils for increased bioavailability, but you could also use olive oil, hempseed oil heck, you could even use butter! Ultimately, it's up to you and how you want to use the finished product. You will extract CBD into the oil using heat and then strain off the plant matter, leaving CBD-enriched oil behind. The resulting oil is much easier to work with than what the alcohol method yields, and there are fewer precautions you need to take throughout the process. To do this, you'll need:

- 1 oz of flower of your choosing, finely ground. We recommend using a grinder, but even chopping up the herb with a knife beforehand is better than nothing. The smaller the pieces you can get the herb into, the more efficiently the CBD will be extracted.
- 16 oz MCT oil, coconut oil, or other oil of your choosing.

A double boiler or crock pot—the key to this method is keeping the heat low, slow, and uniform, allowing the mixture to cook for several hours over indirect, consistent heat without risking it getting too hot and burning all your hard work away.

Utensils—use glass, ceramic, or stainless steel bowls and silicone spatulas for ease, as well as to keep potentially harmful plastics out of your oil.

Step 1: Decarboxylation

Since you've ground the herb up finely, the next step is to decarboxylate, or decarb, the flower, which changes the CBD into its active form, thereby making it more available to the body. To clarify, the CBDA ('A' for acidic) found in dried flowers is in its non-active form; thus, it needs to be decarboxylated into its active form, or what we traditionally think of as CBD. This can be done on a cookie sheet in an oven at 220-225 degrees Fahrenheit for about 60 minutes for maximum conversion. After the time is up, remove the flower from the oven to cool.

Step 2: Extraction

Once you've decarbed the starting material, mix your carrier oil and decarbed flower into the top of a double boiler and place over a pot of simmering (not boiling!) water. Low heat on most stovetops should be sufficient to get the water bath hot enough to extract the CBD without risking scorching the oil. You can also use a crock pot as an alternative to a double boiler.

2-3 hours is sufficient time for the CBD to dissolve into the oil; though, there is no harm in going longer. You don't need to monitor the oil too closely: checking in every half hour or to stir and monitor its color should be sufficient. When it's a deep, earthy brownish green, you'll know it's ready.

After the time is up, pour the oil and flower through some cheesecloth (coffee filters will work in a pinch) to strain off the plant matter, leaving behind the CBD-rich oil. If you're using cheesecloth, be sure to squeeze out all the oil you can from the bundle of plant matter—a potato ricer is super handy for this, but not necessary if you don't mind using a little elbow grease. Discard the leftover starting material, it's work here is done. You can then place the oil in a bottle or jar and store it in a cool, dry place away from the sun and other light sources.

Homemade CBD Oil

Congratulations, you've made your first batch of homemade CBD oil! The resulting oil can be used orally in the form of tinctures or made into gelatin capsules, or even added to food if the taste is unpleasant to you on its own. The oil can also be applied directly to the skin for topical pain relief, added to your favorite body care products before application, or incorporated into your diet a few drops at a time. Its uses are just as versatile as the CBD you would have bought from a retailer, only it's custom-designed by you, for you.

In order to properly dose the CBD oil you just made, you can use our edible potency calculator here. The most important factor will be the amount of CBD contained in your starting material—any reputable supplier will be able to tell you this.

Conclusion

While there are a number of quality CBD oils available for purchase, making a high-quality CBD oil at home is attainable, affordable, and low-risk using the oil infusion method discussed above. Oil extraction uses indirect, low heat to gradually extract CBD without any harsh fumes or flammability precautions. It's the safest and simplest way to supply yourself with homemade CBD oil.

Different Ways on How to Make CBD Oil

Now that we have established the benefits, let us go to the main part of the discussion. To make your own CBD oil, keep in mind the methods that will be mentioned below. Personal preferences, as well as the tools that are available, will dictate the method that will be right for you. Be sure to religiously follow the instructions to maximize the benefits of CBD in the oil that you will make.

Oil Method

With this method, there is a need to choose a carrier oil, such as olive or coconut oil. This is increasing in popularity because it allows the user to take advantage not only of the CBD that is extracted but also of the carrier oil that is going to be used.

Here is how you can make CBD oil through the oil method:

- With the use of a weed grinder, choose buds by bud trimmer, leaves, and stems of a high-quality cannabis plant. The quality of the cannabis that will be used will dictate the quality of the oil that will be produced. Before doing this, however, the parts of the cannabis have to go through a process known as decarboxylation. To do this, you have to bake the buds and leaves at a temperature of 220 degrees Fahrenheit for about 90 to 100 minutes.
- In a mason jar, mix the ground weed with the carrier oil of choice. For the purpose of this guide, we will make one with coconut oil. You have to saturate the weed with the oil. You can reduce the oil or add more depending on how potent you want the end product to be.
- Bring the mixture to a boil. Place the lid of the mason jar and make sure to secure it in place. On the bottom of the pan, place a towel. Place the jar on the top and fill it with water until it reaches a temperature of at least 200 degrees. It will be good if you have a thermometer.
- Leave the pot for about three hours. From time to time, check the pot and see to it that the water has not evaporated. Turn off the stove after three hours and let it sit for another three hours. Heat it

again for three hours, turn off the heat, and leave it for the night.

The next morning, your CBD oil is ready. Strain it using a cheesecloth, squeeze, and your oil is ready to be used as you desire.

Alcohol Method

Also known as the ethanol method, it is another process that does not require special skills or advanced equipment, making it another good choice for beginners thinking of how to make CBD oil. Alcohol is preferred as an extracting agent because it does not leave an unpleasant taste or odor.

- Put the weed in a ceramic or glass bowl. Cover it with alcohol and stir for about 6 minutes. Use a wooden spoon to extract the resin.
- Place a straining bag or sieve to filter the solvent out of the container. Squeeze as much extract as possible. You can repeat the process if you think that you can still extract more oil from weed that you are squeezing.
- In a double boiler, pour the oil that you have earlier extracted. Heat it until bubbles start to form. Wait until the alcohol evaporates but do not raise the temperature. Wait until it simmers in about thirty

minutes while making sure that the flame is low. Once the alcohol evaporates completely, mix it.
- Transfer the concentrated oil in a storage bottle. Be sure to keep the lid tight to avoid damaging its quality and effectiveness.

The Different Ways to Use CBD Oil

Now that you have made you own CBD oil, the next concern would be how to use it. This is one thing that requires careful thought, which will be instrumental in its effectiveness.

- Spray: This is one of the least preferred ways of consumption basically because of the low concentration of CBD oil. You can put the oil in a spray bottle. To use, spray one to three times on the mouth.
- Vaping: The inhalation of CBD oil is one more thing that holds a lot of promise. Using a vape will also provide you with the opportunity to adjust the dosage of the CBD that gets into your body.
- Tinctures: It is known for its purity, which is the reason why it is the most popular way of using CBD oil. All that you have to do is to apply a few drops of CBD oil under the tongue. This is popular as well for the quick absorption for optimal effects.

- Concentrates: If you want a high dosage of CBD extract to be absorbed by the body, this is the method that you should choose. It is believed to be stronger by as much as ten times compared to other forms of using CBD oil.
- Ingestion: The taste of CBD oil can be foul for some people. While you can consume it straight, it can also be used in the form of a capsule that contains CBD oil. With this, you will be able to swallow it without the burden of an unwanted taste.
- Creams: You can also use CBD oil in the form of topical applications. Creams with CBD oil can be used in the treatment of various skin conditions and in providing immediate pain relief.
- Edibles: If you have ever been in a place where weed is legal, you will see a lot of edibles, many of which use CBD oil as the main ingredient. From cookies to gummy bears, people have been creative in thinking of ways how to digest CBD oil

Easy Steps

Step 1: Assemble the ingredients and tools you will need

You will be using are 1 ounce of medical marijuana, available with a California medical marijuana card, and 1 gallon of high proof alcohol, such as Everclear. Be certain to use alcohol that is intended for human consumption, do not use rubbing alcohol.

The tools you will need are 1 medium glass or ceramic mixing bowl, a wooden spoon, a straining device such as a muslin bag, cheesecloth or coffee filter paired with a mesh strainer, a container to catch liquid, a silicon spatula, a double boiler, a plastic syringe, and glass jars. At various stages in the process you will need to wear a respirator mask, non-latex gloves, safety glasses and oven mitts.

Step 2: Extract the cannabinoids from the cannabis

Soak the cannabis buds in the alcohol by putting the MMJ into the ceramic bowl and submerging it in the pure alcohol. Stir and mash the mixture with the wooden spoon for about 3 minutes. Strain the mixture, letting the dark green cannabis infused alcohol pour into the second container while trapping the solid mash in the strainer.

Step 3: Do a second strain

Put the mashed up contents of the strainer back into the first bowl, submerge in fresh alcohol and mix and mash for another 3 minutes. Then strain the new mixture and add the remaining green liquid to the green liquid from the first strain.

Step 4: Fill glass jars or syringes with cannabis oil

Draw the cannabis oil into the plastic syringe by pulling on the plunger. Transfer the oil from the syringe into a clean glass jar with an airtight lid.

Step 5: Store in a cool, dark place

Keep the oil in the airtight glass jars in a cool, dark cabinet. The oil gets hard in cool temperatures, so gently warm the oil to turn it back into liquid before use.

How To Make Cannabis Oil At Home: Rick Simpson's Way

First, gather your ingredients. You will need:

Three to four hours for the process from start to finish.

99.5% Isopropyl Alcohol. Use 2 gallons (7.57 liters) per pound or 2 cups (~500 ml) for an ounce of cannabis. We also suggest chilling your alcohol in a freezer overnight. It will separate the trichomes from the flower more easily.

Marijuana. Rick Simpson will use shake and trim to make topical solutions for skin afflictions. However, he insists that only the choicest, trichome-laden, cannabis indica colas should be used to make Canna Oil for treating cancer. The amount of cannabis oil that each strain can produce will vary, but one ounce of good organic marijuana will typically produce about three to four grams of oil. Rick Simpson's method works best with larger amounts of cannabis.

Next, gather your supplies. You will need:

- Two stainless steel stock pots or food-grade plastic buckets.
- Long wooden stirring spoon or 2×2 piece of chemical-free lumber.
- Stainless steel rice cooker. Caution: A rice cooker with a non-stick surface will leach chemicals into your oil. Stick with stainless steel only.
- A common electric cooling fan and extension cord.
- Plastic funnels.
- Coffee filters.
- Empty clean plastic bottles.
- Stainless steel measuring cup.
- Coffee Warmer.
- Large syringes.

Step #1

Place your weed of choice in a steel pot or food-grade bucket. Dampen the plant matter with chilled isopropyl alcohol (your solvent), and then crush the mixture with a wooden spoon or 2×2 for about five minutes.

Step #2

Add more alcohol until the plant matter is completely immersed. Again, crush and stir the mixture for a further five minute. The crushing action is technically called a "wash" because you are washing the trichomes from plant matter.

NOTE: Trichomes are the resin glands of the cannabis plant. They contain THC, CBD, and other medicinal cannabinoids like CBN, CBG, and CBT. These trichomes are the "thing" that gets you high, cures your insomnia, reduces chronic pain, and may even cure cancer.

Step #3

Block the lip of the pot or bucket with a lid or your 2×2 and slowly pour the solvent into the second bucket. Try to keep as much of the marijuana plant matter in the first bucket for the next step. It's okay if some gets through—you're going to strain it later. But you want as much of the cannabis material left over in the first bucket as possible for the second round of washing.

Step #4

Pour more chilled alcohol into the first bucket until the plant matter is again immersed. Crush the cannabis with your wooden utensil for five more minutes. This step is known as the second wash.

Step #5

Again block the lip of the pot or bucket and slowly pour the solvent from the second wash into the bucket with the solvent from the first wash.

NOTE: The majority of the medicinal resins (75-80%) will be dissolved by the first round of washing. The second round of washing usually dissolves the remaining 20-25%. Because of that, a third round of washing isn't necessary.

If you do choose to do a third round of washing, keep the solvent from that round separate from the first two rounds. The third-round solvent should be used for topical applications, while the first- and second-round solvents should be reserved for ingestion.

Step #6

Leave the solvent to sit while you recycle any leftover plant matter into your compost. Once converted to super soil, you can use it to grow more organic marijuana.

Step #7

Rinse out the first bucket.

Step #8

Place a coffee filter inside a plastic funnel and insert the funnel through the mouth of a small plastic bottle. The size of your straining container will depend on how much solvent you used in the first few steps. You can also use a number of smaller straining containers instead of trying to find one large container.

Pour the mixture in the second bucket through the coffee filters to strain off any excess plant matter. Filter the solvent as many times as it takes to remove all the plant matter.

NOTE: At this point, the solvent will have taken on a dark yellow color. Don't worry. The color comes from the healing resins which are now dissolved in the alcohol. The color and the smell are also influenced by the terpenes that are present on the cannabis plant.

Terpenes are the pungent oils that create the distinct tastes and smells of the numerous pot strains. These flavors can range from sweet and fruity to skunky and earthy to everything in between.

Step #9

Set up the rice cooker and the electric fan outside or in a well-ventilated area.

CAUTION: Make sure that there are no "sparks, open flames, or red-hot elements" in your workspace because the alcohol fumes that you will cook off in your rice cooker are highly flammable and toxic to inhale.

Set up your fan so that it circulates air towards the vents on the bottoms of the rice cooker. See the picture above for a simple illustration of the cooker/fan arrangement. The reason for the fan is that it will prevent the alcohol fumes from condensing to a point where they can ignite.

NOTE: Rick Simpson adds, "I have used this same process hundreds of times and have never had a mishap. But for your own safety, please follow the instructions and make sure the area is well ventilated."

Step #10

Fill the rice cooker as much as three-quarters full with your marijuana solvent mixture. Don't fill the cooker all the way up or it will boil over.

NOTE: At this point, you may be wondering why you are using a rice cooker instead of a crock pot or just a pan and the stove. Rest assured that there's a very good reason for this choice. We'll outline the benefits of the rice cooker before we move on to the next step.

The purpose of the next few steps is basically twofold:

- Separate the alcohol from the dissolved cannabis oil.
- Decarboxylate the cannabis oil.

The vaporization (or boiling) point of isopropyl alcohol (the solvent you used in the first few steps) is around 181°F. The vaporization point of cannabis oil is a little over 300°F. The decarboxylation temperature for cannabis is in the low two hundreds (210-230°F).

Why do you need to know all these numbers? Because you have to maintain just the right temperatures so that your solvent boils off, your oil doesn't, and the leftover oil is decarboxylated.

So why the rice cooker? Rice cookers are automatically set to maintain temperatures in the decarboxylation sweet spot. These temperatures are enough to get your solvent boiling but not enough to vaporize the oil. Crock pots often exceed 300°F and a pot on the stove can be difficult to maintain a consistent low two-hundreds.

Now that you know why you're using a rice cooker, we can move on to the actual separation process.

Step #11

Set the rice cooker to its highest setting to boil off the alcohol solvent. Be sure the fan is running and is aimed at the rice cooker so the alcohol fumes don't condense and explode.

Step #12

As the liquid level in the rice cooker drops, pour in any remaining solvent but don't exceed three-quarters full. This step depends on how big your rice cooker is and how much solvent you produced in the first few steps of the process. If you only have a small amount, you may not need to keep adding solvent.

Step #13

When you're done adding remaining solvent to the rice cooker, and the level in the cooker is reduced to about two inches, add ten to twelve drops of water to mix. The water will help the remaining solvent boil off and will cleanse the oil of solvent residue.

Step #14

Hold the rice cooker with oven mitts and swirl it's oily contents while the last traces of alcohol boil completely off.

Step #15

When the process is near completion, you will notice three things:

- The leftover oil will emit a crackling sound.
- The oil will begin to bubble (that's the source of the crackling sound).
- Steam will start to escape from the oil. It may look like smoke, but don't worry, it's dark steam.
- When those three criteria are satisfied, the separation process is almost done.

Step #16

Wait for the rice cooker to switch to the low setting and then turn it off.

Step #17

Let your fresh cannaoil mixture cool for about five minutes.

NOTE: Rick recommends that you proceed with the next step even though some strains of cannabis can produce an oil that is finished and ready to use at this point.

Step #18

Pour the mixture into a stainless steel measuring cup, and place the cup on a coffee warmer to completely remove any water remaining in the mixture.

This process can take anywhere from a few minutes to an hour or more. It all depends on the terpenes and flavonoids found in the strain you used to make your oil. The terpenes and flavonoids can cause the oil on the coffee warmer to bubble for quite some time.

Step #19

You know the water has been vaporized when all bubbling has ceased. Remove the measuring cup from the coffee warmer and set it aside to cool.

Some oily residue will remain behind in the measuring cup and the rice cooker. There are a number of options for dealing with these leftovers.

You can soak it up with a piece of bread and consume it as medicine later. Keep in mind that the effects of edibles can take an hour or more to kick in. Be careful how much oil-soaked bread you consume.

Wash the cup or the pot with a small amount of alcohol. This creates a hemp oil tincture that varies in medicinal value depending on the amount of oil the alcohol contains. You can use the isopropyl alcohol you used in the first few steps, but don't drink this mixture. Use the isopropyl alcohol tincture on your skin instead. For a tincture you can ingest, wash the rice cooker with a small amount of high-proof drinking alcohol like vodka or Everclear.

Leave the leftovers in the rice cooker for the next time you make cannabis oil. Mixing the oils from different strains can have many beneficial medicinal effects.

Place a small amount of loose tobacco in the rice cooker and heat until the oil is absorbed. The cannabis oil reduces many of the harmful properties contained in the tobacco.

Step #20

After the oil has cooled, draw the warm mixture up into large needleless syringes and allow the mixture to cool into a thick grease like substance that you can easily squeeze out of the syringe. Place the syringe in a cup of hot water if you have trouble squeezing it out after it has cooled.

If you're not going to use your cannabis oil right away, store it in a dark bottle with a lid or a stainless steel container and place that container in a dark, cool place. This keeps air and sunlight from damaging your valuable creation and helps the oil maintain its medical potency for a long time.

"At first, it may seem daunting for some to try to produce their own medicine," Rick Simpson says. But in reality, the process is extremely simple. Simpson also strongly suggests mixing your favorite varieties of good indica-dominant buds to make your own custom marijuana miracle potions.

Cannabis Oil Applications

Topical Uses

You can apply Rick Simpson's cannaoil to any skin affliction. Apply the oil directly to skin cancers, cover with a bandage, and reapply and rebandage every four days until the cancer disappears.

Continue the treatment for two more weeks to completely heal any cancer cells which could remain. "I have never seen a skin cancer return if my instructions are followed," Rick says.

You can also try mixing your cannabis oil with coconut oil and use the concoction for general daily skin health. This mix of cannabis and coconut oil can turn your skin green for a bit depending on how well you made the cannabis oil. Don't worry though, it will wash off.

To keep this green tinge from becoming a problem, you could apply the oil at night and then scrub it off in the morning when you shower.

Edible Uses

Cannabis oil is much more concentrated than regular cannabis products like the bud you smoke. For that reason, it's best to start small and work your way up from there.

Rick Simpson suggests 1 gram (or 1 ml) of homemade cannabis oil as a full dose. One gram of cannabis oil looks like a pile of about 16 to 8 grains of dry short-grain rice. But again, before you run out and down a gram of cannabis oil, Rick recommends starting small.

In general, he says, it takes new users about 90 days to work up to ingesting the full treatment without getting dysfunctionally high.

That's why Simpson starts new patients off with a serving size that looks like half a dry grain of rice. That may seem tiny and inconsequential, but remember, cannabis oil is quite a bit more concentrated than other cannabis products.

Start off taking this half-a-dry-grain-of-rice serving three times a day. An easy schedule to follow is:

- First thing in the morning with breakfast
- In the afternoon after lunch
- About an hour before you go to sleep

Follow this dosage for four days, then double the dosage to the size of a full grain of rice for the next four days (see the chart above). Rick typically doubles the dosage for patients every four days until they reach the full amount.

Taking the full dose head on without titrating (building up to it) will certainly not kill you. Indeed, some of his patients report enjoying the full dose right off the bat. And Simpson has seen brand new patients with no 420 fears take the full dose first thing.

Many of these patients are declared completely cancer-free just one month after beginning the full dose. According to Simpson, "The name of the game," in terms of actually ingesting the dose, "is to simply get the oil into the patient's body in the easiest and most pleasant way possible."

Dosage Methods

One of the many nice things about cannabis oil is that you can take it in a variety of ways. Below, we describe some of the most common (and easiest) ways to consume cannabis oil.

Ingest It Directly

The simplest way to consume your cannabis oil is to place it directly on top of your tongue and let it dissolve. You can also place it under your tongue and let it dissolve down your throat.

If you don't like the taste, you can also smear the oil on a piece of bread or in between two pieces of fruit (we like banana) to avoid the taste. You could also try mixing it in your favorite drink to make it easier to consume.

Ingesting the cannabis oil in this way should give you the strong kind of 11-Hydroxy-THC body high with an onset that can take up to two hours. If you're familiar with edibles, this is the same thing.

Place It Under Your Tongue (Sublingual)

Another way to consume your cannabis oil is to dab the cannaoil under your tongue and let it dissolve into your bloodstream through your sublingual artery. This method produces effects a little bit faster than ingesting it. The results will be akin to a heady marijuana tincture high.

Vaporize It

You can also vaporize cannabis oil in a vape pen. This is an extremely easy way to take your cannabis oil with you wherever you go. Simply fill up the vape pen's chamber with your homemade oil, and you're ready to go anytime.

Dab It

Another great way to consume cannabis oil is to dab it on a rig like a concentrate. Dabbing a bit of cannabis oil is one of the quickest ways to feel the effects.

When you vaporize the cannabis oil, as you do when you dab, the vapor is absorbed much more quickly into your bloodstream and reaches your brain much sooner than it would if you ingest it.

You will, of course, need a special dabbing rig, but the initial outlay of money is well worth it for the fast-acting high or pain relief you can achieve.

Smoke It

And, of course, you can always rely on the old tried-and-true method of consuming cannabis products: you can smoke it. How do you smoke an oil?

Like this. For a truly out-of-this-world experience, we highly recommend first glazing a joint of your favorite marijuana strain in cannabis oil. Then, cover the whole thing in kief crystals. The resulting combination is a stone cold recreational high! Just be careful. This much ganja goodness in one place can take you on a truly transcendental trip.

Summary

Cannabis oil is one of the purest forms of medicinal cannabis. Homemade oil made from marijuana saved Rick Simpson from a debilitating head injury and from skin cancer.

Cannabis oil is incredibly versatile as it can be applied topically, ingested, or inhaled. Simpson saved thousands of people from a myriad of maladies with nothing more than some simple materials and some really good marijuana. Honestly, you can too!

How to make cannabis cooking oil or cannabis butter with already-vaped weed

Use the weed you just vaporized to make a base ingredient for treats to maintain a longer high. You'll need the following ingredients and tools:

- ½-ounce weed from your vaporizer
- ½-cup of oil (olive, coconut, or canola) or ½-cup of unsalted butter
- Medium-size sauce pan
- Wooden spoon or spatula
- Cheesecloth for straining, or a coffee filter
- Container for storing what you've made

- Make a sort of tea bag with the weed inside the cheesecloth or coffee filter. Put the oil or butter in the sauce pan with the bag.
- Heat this mixture on low until it starts to simmer, or bubble just a little bit. Keep it going while you stir it off and on for 20 minutes.
- Let it cool a bit and squeeze all the oil or butter out of the bag. Pour your new special oil into a container.
- Now, go make brownies or cookies or whatever you like, using your new cannabis oil to add a zing to your meal.

Besides this quick and easy recipe, here's another variation:

- Cannabis cooking oil version 2: with fresh weed
- For this recipe use weed that has not been vaped. You'll want to grind it up.

Once it's ground, here's how to make cannabis oil with it:

- Select an oil to use: coconut and canola are great for desserts while olive oil is good for salads and sautéing veggies. Canola tolerates high heat better than the other two oils.

- Measure out a ratio of two parts oil to one part cannabis.
- Heat the mixture on low to activate the THC without destroying it. You can heat it in one of three different ways—in a saucepan for at least three hours while stirring frequently, in a double-boiler for six to eight hours, or in a crockpot on low for six hours or up to three days.
- Once you're done cooking it, strain the oil with a coffee filter, cheesecloth, or even just a strainer if it wasn't ground too small. Then store it in an odor-free container. It will keep fresh up to two months, or longer in the refrigerator.
- That concludes our section on how to make cannabis oil for cooking. Now we're about to explore making essential oil with cannabis. It's a powerful cure for cancer among other things.

How to make cannabis oil for medical purposes

Making your own essential oil from cannabis isn't the same as making Butane Hash Oil (BHO) because you'll be using alcohol instead of a more dangerous solvent. Still, be careful. Make it in a well-ventilated area and don't exceed the recommended cooking temperatures.

Tools and ingredients needed
- 1 ounce of marijuana, preferably a strain high in THC (Alternatively, you can use two to three ounces of medical marijuana trim)
- 1 gallon of Everclear or 99% pure ETHYL/ETHANOL alcohol
- Stock pot or food safe container large enough to hold the gallon of alcohol and marijuana
- Wooden spoon for stirring
- Bubble hash bags for straining, specifically a 73 micron bag
- A double boiler makes the boiling process a lot easier than using a single pot or pan, but do not use one with a Teflon coating because it leeches chemicals
- Containers or syringes to store the oil when you're done

Make the oil

You can make your own medical cannabis oil in a weekend.

- Start by putting alcohol in the pot, then submerging the marijuana in the alcohol. Put that in the freezer overnight. The alcohol won't freeze but the cold will help extract the resin.

- The next morning, take the pot out of the freezer. Use the wooden spoon to gently stir without smashing the flowers.
- Strain the mixture through the bubble hash bag (the 73-micron weave). Repeat the rinse with fresh alcohol.
- Now place the alcohol with cannabis essence into the double boiler. Let the double boiler boil off all the alcohol. Be careful because the alcohol fumes will be VERY strong. It's best to do this outdoors if at all possible. At the least, turn on a fan and open windows. While boiling, check the temperature to make sure it stays at least 212 degrees F (100 C) and below 290 degrees F (140 C) for 75 minutes. That way the THC is activated but not ruined. Tip: use a reliable thermometer.
- When you're done boiling off the alcohol, you'll see an oily substance at the bottom of the pan. Pour that into a glass container or into syringes if you like. Store it in a cool, dark place. If it gets hard, gently warm it up with warm water.

Why make your own cannabis oil for medical purposes

Have you ever heard of the Canadian guy named Rick Simpson? He was diagnosed with skin cancer but healed himself in a matter of days with cannabis oil. He believed in the stuff so much that he made it and gave it away for free. This of course resulted in raids by the Canadian Mounted Police. Rick and his family moved to Europe to a place where he can enjoy marijuana without prosecution.

People have benefited from using cannabis oil to treat conditions like cancer, chronic pain, epilepsy, and PTSD. They may consume between one to three drops a day or they place the oil directly on their skin, depending on the situation.

Another person who seems to have cured his own cancer with cannabis oil is a retired man from Great Britain. He had a liver transplant to ward off cancer, but then the cancer attacked his new organ. He found a video online that inspired him to try cannabis oil. Within three days his pain was gone. His biopsy found no cancer in his new liver.

Made in the USA
Lexington, KY
07 August 2019